7 - DAY FULL-BODY DETOX DIET GUIDE

Cleanse your liver, lungs, kidney, skin,

Using Dr. Sebi Intra-Cellular Cleansing Method for Rapid Weight Loss, Improved Health, Stop Disease, and Reverse Aging.

Contents

Introduction

Why is Dr. Sebi Intra-Cellular Cleansing Necessary?

Chapter One

Reasons to Detox Using Dr. Sebi Intra-Cellular Cleansing Methods

Common Poisonous substances Around Us

Chapter 2

A Guide for the Selection of Complementary and Alternative Remedial Therapies

Getting Started

Precautions and What to Expect During Detoxification

Chapter 3

The Dr. Sebi 7 Day Detox Round-up

First Simple Practice

Second Simple Practice

Entire Detox Week

Chapter 4

The Dr. Sebi 7 Day Plan – A Day by Day Intra-Cellular Detox Formula

Day 1 and Day 2

Day 3

Day 4

Day 5

Days 6 and 7

Chapter 5

Dr. Sebi Alkaline/Electric Food Recipes (Directions for Detox)

Dr. Sebi Life-giving or Vitalizing Beverages

Dr. Sebi Superfoods Detox Broth Recipes

Dr. Sebi Smoothie Recipes

Digestive Tea or CCF Tea

Hearty Vegetarian Chili Recipe – Makes 7-10 Servings

Simple Soup Recipe – 4 – 6 Servings

Chapter 6

Dr. Sebi Herbs to Detox the Liver.

Related Books to Buy by the Same Author

Introduction

Welcome to Dr. Sebi Full Body Detox Guide – Cleanse Yourself from Bad Habits Using Dr. Sebi Intra – Cellular Cleansing Methods.

When cleansing the body with respect to Dr. Sebi's intra-cellular method, most people are doing it for the first time after a long time of bad living habits. Before getting started, you should know that to cleanse and repair your body successfully, your emotional mind must also be in a correct state alongside the willpower to change what you consume at the moment.

According to Dr. Sebi, Intra Cellular cleansing is a cleansing process that ensures proper nourishment and strengthening of the cell, alongside cleaning the entire matrix of the cell or cells that make up the full body system.

Why is Dr. Sebi Intra-Cellular Cleansing Necessary?

The process is designed to break into bits the calcification, toxins, acids, and mucus that has accumulated in the body over the years.

The Organs and Systems to Be Cleansed

- Colon

- Lymphatic System

- Skin

- Liver

- Kidneys

- Lungs

Now looking at the Bio-Electric Cell Food: Intra-Cellular Cleansing Guide, we will help you draw out a perfect 7-Day Detox guide that will help your body get rid of mucus that have been accumulated over the years.

Ready to reverse your age, lose weight, and improve your general well-being?

Make sure you stick to this Seven Days Detox Plan and avoid all that needs to be avoided.

Chapter One

Reasons to Detox Using Dr. Sebi Intra-Cellular Cleansing Methods

Many a times, people question why we must use Dr. Sebi method to detoxify the body. Well, if you've read my other books, you'd have definitely understood the reason.

This is a working method with lots of testimonies from users all over the world. If it works for them, it should also work for you!

Generally, detoxification is a treatment for poisoning done by neutralizing the toxic properties in our body. It could also be a treatment for drug and alcoholic addiction. From a drug and alcohol perspective, detoxifying the body works by removing, or it is merely the removal of the physiological effects duly caused by addictiveness to harmful substances. These hazardous substances are not toxic drugs and other bruising substances. It could be as a result of the toxic-filled environment that we dwell in. This implies that detoxification merely is various poisons removal.

The world today is filled or occupied by various harmful substances. These are often as a result of men crave and the great desire for mind-blowing innovations, high-level technology and much more. Even though these creations or debuts ease our lives, they sadly arrive with ill sides, and these activities are barely communicated to the unsuspecting public. The exposed persons, therefore, suffer the consequences of the situation with severe health-related issues bandaging their necks.

It's time to set your body free from

Common Poisonous substances Around Us

- **Manufactured toxins** such as Sarin and dioxin

- **Toxins from bacteria** around our environment and we have the likes of Clostridium botulinum

- **Improper use of medications** which are often termed drug abuse

- **Allergens** from various unsuspicious chemicals

- **Mushrooms** equally infect with toxins, and we have Muscarine from poisonous mushrooms like the *death cap* and the *fool's mushroom*

- **Foreign substances** like metals, and even medicines

- **Microbial toxins** caused by micro-organisms including bacteria and fungi. An example is Botulinum and other virile toxins.

Apart from viruses or bacteria-related toxins, there are other forms of toxins that are attributed to emotions. Emotional toxins are hazardous to human health. They create some kind of mental instability in the brains thereby causing the victim to lose self-consciousness at that period.

- **Habitual dissatisfaction** like always complaining about things even if there is no better way to achieve them

- **Damaging emotions** that can admonish detrimental thoughts and actions which often lead to unnecessary wailings

- **Extreme anxiety** such that we bask in a relatively permanent state of worry and nervousness which can as well deny any form openness

- **Concurrent low self-esteem** like harboring thoughts that makes you feel undesirable and useless

- **Toxic anger** always raged over nothing. Certain unnecessary things ignite inflamed furiousness at all times.

- **Keeping incessant grudges**, bearing ill feelings that do not encourage positivity towards a person or activity in question

- **Depression,** a sunken mood, sad feeling of gloom and sever sense of inadequacy and often lead to regrettable circumstances

- **Aching noise** usually from open places leaves the mind destabilized and unfocused. It is worse when it happens almost all the time.

Despite these negative mental demanding situations being undesirable and defective, we still have the upper hand when it comes to sweeping them under the carpet. The human body is programmed in such a way that the various organs can operate to ensure a state of equilibrium in our all-around emotional states.

When the human body can operate with some level of metabolic equilibrium, it is called homeostasis. Various principal body systems work together to achieve this equilibrium, and they include:

- The skin

- The Lungs

- The brain

- Immune system

- Kidney

- The muscular, skeletal system and nervous system

- Stomach

- Sternum (breastbone)

Sometimes detoxification may malfunction in your body due to various reasons. No particular symptom can be used to decipher when the natural detoxification of our organs is not working. When these natural detoxifications in our body system fail, it might lead to severe damage to the body system. But then, certain possible things could serve as a determinant for the failure of detoxification in your body.

- Joints pain

- Bloating and gas

- Bowel disruption

- Headaches and restlessness

- Sexual insensitivity

- Sores and body rashes

- Irritation of the skin

- Sterility

- Weight loss

- Loss of muscle and weakness

- Vascular illnesses

- Persistent mood swings

- Stomach cramps

- Bad breath and body odor

- Nervousness and metal instability

- Sinus congestion

- Craving for food

This short manual has been put up to defend the usefulness of various detoxification therapies. These therapies will considerably substitute for the failure of your body system to detoxify. One might be left basking in significant dysphoria. This is because of the fear that the body is at this point vulnerable due to its inability to detoxify in conformity to how it is being programmed to function. But not to worry, detoxification therapy is good to do mean of compensating the difficulties. Despite these therapies being useful, there are still harmful ones out there. Such that can roughly alter your body or worsen the situation, as the case may be. This is sometimes due to how some manufacturers go as far as over-enlarging beyond bounds, the effectiveness of their product. It may be difficult to know which is good and which is wrong but then, making thorough research and reading reviews of specific therapies provided by certain untrusted or unknown manufacturers will significantly help to bring about the best option to your way.

In any standard detoxification program, specific components are very necessary and as a result, must not be omitted. This should include but not limited to.

Hydration – One healthy way is to cleanse the cells with water. This action can be easily reversed where necessary. You should have a reasonable intake of water daily.

Regular Exercise – Exercise, even before any detoxification program is a necessary activity that ensures healthy living. A standard detoxification program should include this aspect as the most important if not necessary activity. A simple bench press or workout should suffice.

Nutriment – The intake of specific food containing required food nutrients.

Rest and Timed Sleep – While resting, your body feels more relax and it initiates some form of refreshment to the system. Resting is always the best way to end any detoxification program as it aids in the repair of the body system.

Chapter 2

A Guide for the Selection of Complementary and Alternative Remedial Therapies

Detoxification as a complementary and alternative kind of therapy helps your body to heal and regain itself instead of conducting a conventional medical treatment. It can be done or used side by side with conventional medicine as well.

Before thinking of this option, there are questions you must be sure to have answers to.

➤ Will detoxing solve the problem?

➤ Is this form of treatment safe?

➤ How well will this treatment deal with my problem and what should I anticipate?

➤ How can I pick the right detox?

➤ Does my condition or body system support?

➤ How much is this form of treatment, can I afford it?

➤ What are the benefits of detoxification?

Several approaches can be used to detox the body. Of these approaches, it is not quite easy to tell which is superior to the other. This is because all the detox approaches tend to proffer positive or reliable results if used done accurately. This notwithstanding, having a 7-day steadfast to certain activities with guaranteed health boost will be a better fit for the occasion. This manual will provide you with a simple and easy-to-follow guide that will assist in detoxifying yourself.

Getting Started

This systematic plan for therapy is designed to serve a particular purpose and not to be taken as an all-in-one guide. This short manual is projected to be a useful companion, and a perfect health aiding guide. If necessary, it can be altered to suit the required or newly specified function. Since the detoxification course does not require any form of planning, nor preparation, it will be best to go through and mastermind yourself with this guide before time.

1. This guide equally stresses the mental relation with the body. It dialects basically on the natural approaches which in most cases help to alleviate faulted mental processes. It also disentangles the adverse effects that result in emotional distress.

2. One of the most important things to note in a detox program is to sort out reasons that define why you are into it. It is equally advisable to keep to your expectations to avoid being disappointed with the outcome. If possible, bring up reasons by peening down justifications for your opting into detoxification. Put up ideas that will encourage you.

3. There are several essential components of detoxification. These, if followed will boost and help the body to build up activities that will enable it to heal. These activities are not restricted to anyone, and it is a rather cool idea for you to initiate it with your body. You can always get medical pieces of advice that will help you to know how beneficial it will be for you.

4. They are making use of excellent and effective methods of detoxification matters a lot. These methods may often time be costly in terms of its requirements, but it's worth every bit.

Precautions and What to Expect During Detoxification

Opting for the right detox program is essential. Making enquiries helps to determine which is better for you.

➢ During the detoxification regimen, certain unstable situations posing extreme danger or difficulty may occur. These occurrences are mostly health-related and might alter the whole process. This being said, there are some common signs or symptoms that popup during detoxification and they include: mood swing, severe headache, joints weakness, fatigue, gas and bloating, skin irritation, restlessness, difficulty in concentrating, skin problems, cravings and irritability and moodiness. The appearance of these symptoms is often determined by several conditions including sugar level (low or high sugar level), body response to the environment, and disengagement from negatively effective drugs and so on.

➢ Keeping easily accessible or in close contact with your medical doctor or clinical psychologist is necessary in case of an emergency. You will also have to frequently converse with them and be sure that there is a follow-up of your detox by the doctor.

➢ The dangers of self-guided detoxification are still there. You should remain strictly under medical supervision to avoid health complications.

➢ Developing any of these symptoms suggests that there should be a keep up with the detox process. But in the case of emergency or circumstances of psychological suffering from the activity, it is best to discontinue.

➢ Water is necessary while on this course. Dehydrating makes a good and plausible option.

➢ Be sure to follow and make use of only the prescribed form of treatments and medication daily.

Following up this short guide the way it will provide a positive and required result from the detox.

Chapter 3

The Dr. Sebi 7 Day Detox Round-up

First Simple Practice

* **Day 1 & Day 2** – Avoid certain foods like meat, chocolate, and any other food that contains sugar. Make use of lemon juice to wash and cleanse your body system. The lemon is best when squeezed and taken in a cup of hot water. If you are not a vegetarian, you should make yourself one at the moment. You should exercise for at least an hour during these days. And keep going with the intake of vegetal foods.

* **Day 3** – you should still avoid the intake of any meat. Raw food is the most preferable on this day, and you can try to exercise your mind, i.e., detox your emotions. You

can do this by observing some minutes of about 18 - 25 minutes of meditation. Avoid eating grains at the moment.

* **Day 4** – Plenty water intake, otherwise called hydration. Anything watery will do but be mindful of sugary drinks. And stop the intake of vegetal foods for this day.

* **Day 5** – Repeat what you have on day **1** and this time, you may eat raw vegetables but in small quantities.

* **Day 6 & Day 7** – Repeat day 3 activities, meditate for some time and drink water from time to time. Ensure the continuation of a period without meat. Follow and repeat what you have on day **1** and day **2**.

Second Simple Practice

This other detox practice can suffice for detox of 7 days or more.

- Have your lemon around. Squeeze and drink to cleanse your body system and also eat vegetal foods and fruits as well.

- Make time to exercise your body at regular intervals.

- Water should be your partner at the moment. Ensure that you have a decent amount of water intake regularly.

- You can keep records to keep track of your activities.

- Remember that emotions can be toxic as well. Perform metal detox.

Entire Detox Week

There are several necessary things you need to do during the whole week of detox to boost or aid your body throughout the detox week. These include getting rid of fatty foods like mackerel, snail, chicken, pork, and others.

Also, avoid foods with sugary components or sugar. Anything that tastes like sugar or sweetener must be avoided during this period. For more detox effectiveness, avoid the intake of alcohol or any alcoholic substance either for recreation or for any other reason at all.

Exercise your body to trigger sweat. It is okay to sweat as it will help to expel some of the toxins from your body. Drink more water and urinate when you are pressed. Avoid egg and continue with vegetal foods and fruits.

Chapter 4

The Dr. Sebi 7 Day Plan – A Day by Day Intra-Cellular Detox Formula

Day 1 and Day 2

It is recommended that you make available vegetal foods on days **1** and **2**. The vegetable can either be fresh vegetable or frozen. Neither of the two does not matter. In case you are following the **first simple practice**, drinking naturally squeezed lemon juice and cereals or grains intake are highly recommended.

Other advisable things to do include:

- ✓ Making use of foodstuffs grown or raised without synthetic fertilizers. The foods can be cold pressed with extra virgin olive oil.

- ✓ This can be flavored with the addition of healthy aromatic vegetable substances like spices.

- ✓ Drink tea all day, especially minted tea. It will help to increase bile secretion and encourage bile flow, which helps to speed and ease digestion.
- ✓ Take in well-filtered water of about 6 to 11 glassfuls. Top this up with smoothies and diluted juices. The sugar strength if present must be very low.
- ✓ Have mixed nuts, vegetables and fruits for noshes or snacks.
- ✓ Make use of herbal dosing to help in the days' treatment. The herb would be best if it's recommended.
- ✓ You should put in about an hour or half an hour of exercise. It could be jogging, a long walk, bicycling, jumping, and so on.

- ✓ Make it customary of yourself to address and detox your mental self. Take a deep breath as well as some minutes of meditation.
- ✓ Having steam room therapy will have beneficial effects on your cardiovascular system. You should consider this as an option.
- ✓ Get some rest. This should relax your body and refresh your entire body system.

Day 3

You should eliminate any form of meat on Day 3. Do away with rice, beans, and any non-vegetal edibles. You should take, even in a more significant amount, vegetables, and fruits. The vegetables should be healthily prepared, and the fruits must be well washed and frozen, if possible. You can equally introduce some practices in Days 1 and 2.

- ✓ Virgin olive oil

- ✓ Healthy aromatic vegetable substance like spices and seasonings as well
- ✓ Herbal supplements intake (optional)
- ✓ Carry out an abstemious exercise of your body.
- ✓ Drink well-filtered water, diluted juice, and even smoothies
- ✓ Get some rest and try to meditate.
- ✓ Take in minted tea.

Additionally, massage therapy is recommended on Day **3**. Massage therapy manually manipulates the body and relaxes the entire body system.

Day 4

At this point, you should disassociate yourself from any solid food. Hydrate your body by drinking a lot of water and diluted juices and even smoothies. In Day **4**, it is imperative to be attentive to your body for any changes. You can also consider.

- ✓ Plenty intake of tea with less sugar

- ✓ Rest enough and relax your bones. Do not exercise and if at all you feel it is necessary to exercise you are to avoid heavy workouts.

- ✓ A quick nap and meditate for like 15 – 20 minutes.

- ✓ Unlike in the second point of this list, avoid hard work. If you must do anything, it should be very minimal or take the least possible action.

- ✓ Take in lots of fluids to help hydrate and regulate your body system.

Bowel Cleansing Regimen (Optional)

- ➢ On this day of reduced or no food intake, you should take Bentonite Clay of about 500 – 1000 mg. You may opt for Activated Charcoal Capsules, and this should be done orally. This should be taken three times per day. This is one good way to detoxify.

➤ For bowel elimination, you should drink 300 mL of Magnesium Citrate in the morning.

➤ For bowel elimination in the afternoon, take about 1 – 2 saline Fleet Enemas.

Day 5 (This practice will be the same as in Day 3)

This day is when you reintroduce fruits, vegetables, and other vegetal foods. Take them in any quantity that suits you. You can have them frozen, dried, or fresh. Be sure to prepare them healthily so that it will support the body tissues. You do not require any unique or new activity on this day. All you need now is to reinvent the operations in Days **1** to **3**.

- ✓ Olive oil
- ✓ Healthy aromatic vegetable substance like spices and seasonings
- ✓ You can retake the herbal medications now, but it is optional.
- ✓ Have a light exercise which you did not on Day **4**
- ✓ Journaling or medication
- ✓ Drink well-filtered water, diluted juice, and even smoothies

✓ Get some rest and try to meditate.

✓ Have mixed nuts, vegetables and fruits for noshes or snacks.

✓ Have steam room therapy for the benefit of your cardiovascular system.

You can equally include energy work sessions to help relax and balance your body system.

Days 6 and 7 (Similar to Days 1 and 2)

You can also collect mushrooms, legumes, beans, and several other healthy grains. Continue with the intake of vegetal foods. The below-mentioned activities are also recommended.

✓ Use virgin olive oil.

✓ Healthy aromatic vegetable substances like spices and healthy seasonings

✓ Perform light exercises.

- ✓ Drink well-filtered water, mixed juice, and even smoothies' healthy smoothies.
- ✓ Take mixed nuts, vegetables and fruits for noshes or snacks.
- ✓ Have steam room therapy for the benefit of your cardiovascular system.
- ✓ Journaling or medication
- ✓ Have mixed nuts, vegetables and fruits for noshes or snacks.

Chapter 5

Dr. Sebi Alkaline/Electric Food Recipes (Directions for Detox)

Dr. Sebi Life-giving or Vitalizing Beverages

Since Day **4** was more like a fasting period, this will make an excellent option for intake.

- ✓ About 1 – 2 tablespoonful of real maple syrup
- ✓ Including a tablespoon or two tablespoons of fresh lemon. You can equally opt for lime juice.
- ✓ A small pinch of Cayenne pepper
- ✓ Distilled water

The glass to be used should not be short. It should be a tall glass so that it can contain the syrup, juice and Cayenne to be combined. Also recommended is diluted fruit juice.

Dr. Sebi Superfoods Detox Broth Recipes

Superfoods Detox Broth is very useful, mainly if you use foodstuffs grown or raised without synthetic fertilizers oz the likes. It will make a decent companion on Day **4**, and it will help principally in detoxing your body during the course.

- ✓ A medium-sized pot
- ✓ A big bowl and a filter for the soup
- ✓ Two medium carrots
- ✓ Three stalks of sliced celery
- ✓ Japanese sweet potato
- ✓ A chopped onion
- ✓ A handful of fresh parsley leaves
- ✓ One large piece of seaweed (kombu)
- ✓ Three chopped carrots
- ✓ A grated 1 or 2-inch piece of fresh ginger
- ✓ ½ teaspoon of fine sea salt for better taste

- ✓ Peeled daikon roots.

- ✓ Two stalks of peeled burdock root

- ✓ 3 quarts 1/2 cups water

- ✓ 1 tablespoon of ground turmeric

- ✓ Garlic and bell pepper

Ensure that all the above-listed ingredients are added to the pot. After boiling for about 45 – 60 minutes, fit in your strain in a clean bowl and pour in the cooked items to filter the big particles from the liquid. At this point, your broth is almost ready. Pour in a decent amount of sea salt to add taste to it. Make sure that the food is stored in a well-covered container. You are free to refrigerate it. You are to take this for all days of the detox week and especially on Day **4** when you have to do very little or nothing.

Dr. Sebi Smoothie Recipes

This recipe makes better sense when taken in the morning and the evening. It should amount to about a liter or two. Make use of simple and healthy ingredients.

- ✓ 1/2 frozen banana
- ✓ 1/2 fresh or frozen cup pineapple
- ✓ 1/2 avocado
- ✓ 1/2 unsweetened group yoghurt
- ✓ 1/2 cup of orange juice
- ✓ 7 – 11 ice cubes
- ✓ One organic apple
- ✓ A pear with peel
- ✓ 1/2 cup of mango
- ✓ About three tablespoonfuls of flax seed
- ✓ Flavored milk
- ✓ Spinach
- ✓ Healthy blueberry

The best way to smooth these ingredients is to conflate them using a blender. After the blending, your smoothie is ready for use. The thirst for the smoothie will not be determined by how you mix these ingredients but by how well you can originate ideas that will spice it up. The amount of water to be added depends on the size and number of ingredients used. Add water to the desired quantity. Store in a refrigerator for prolonged quality and good taste.

Digestive Tea or CCF Tea

This is a traditional Ayurvedic remedy. It is called CCF tea, i.e., Coriander-Cumin-Fennel Tea

- ✓ 1/4 tablespoon Coriander
- ✓ 1/4 tablespoon Cumin
- ✓ 1/4 tablespoon Fennel
- ✓ 2 to 3 cups of water

Allow the seeds to simmer for about 5 – 10 minutes. Strain the CCF Tea and use after every meal daily throughout the detox week.

Hearty Vegetarian Chili Recipe – Makes 7-10 Servings

You should make use of simple, healthy, and natural ingredients. Where possible, avoid foodstuffs grown with synthetic fertilizers.

- 5 – 6 cups of well-filtered water
- One tablespoon olive oil
- 1/2 chopped baby Portobello mushroom.
- Sun-dried tomatoes
- One large-chopped onion.
- Three bouillon cubes
- Chilli powder
- One tablespoon of dry parsley

- Four minced gloves garlic

- A chopped zucchini

- 1/2 vegetable broth

- One chopped yellow squash

- One bay leaf

- One can of garbanzo beans

- One tablespoon of ground cumin

- Can tomato sauce.

- A Tablespoon of orange peel

- Salt and pepper (bell pepper) to add taste.

First, fry the mushroom, onions, and the sun-dried tomatoes in olive oil. Stop the brief frying when it becomes tender. And then boil the water and add bouillon to it. Now, remove the sauce mushroom, onions, and sun-dried tomatoes from the cooking pan. You can now mix and stir the sauce or fried mushroom, onions and sun-dried tomatoes with the chili powder, minced garlic, zucchini, yellow squash, dry parsley, bay leaf, garbanzo beans, ground cumin and also the tomato sauce. Simmer for about 10 – 15 minutes until all vegetables or vegetal foods become tender. Your hearty vegetarian chilli is now ready, stored in a refrigerator or the same used cooking pot.

Simple Soup Recipe – 4 – 6 Servings

Make use of simple, healthy, and natural ingredients. Where possible, avoid foodstuffs grown with synthetic fertilizers. There are various kinds of simple soup, and these are the recipes for the Spicy Carrot Soup.

- ➢ A medium-sized cooking pot
- ➢ Three tablespoons of vegetable oil or opt for a cold pressed virgin oil
- ➢ One finely chopped onion or leek
- ➢ A cup of strained barley
- ➢ One deseeded and finely chopped chilli

- Four finely grated or roughly chopped carrots (non-synthetic)

- A pinch of powdered ginger

- One bay leaf

- One vegetable bouillon cube

- Salt and pepper to add taste.

- About 6 – 7 cups of water

Pour oil, barley, and onion after a minute into the saucepan or cooking pot and allow simmering for about 4 – 6 minutes. Add chopped chilli, carrots, powdered ginger, bay leaf, bouillon cube. Cook for five more minutes and stir from time to time. Add salt and pepper or season it to add taste. After this, allow it to simmer for the next 40 minutes. Check and be sure that the carrot is soft and then puree your soup. It is now ready to be served. Store the remaining in a well-covered container or refrigerate it.

Chapter 6

Dr. Sebi Herbs to Detox the Liver.

Dandelion

Dandelion comes in capsule or liquid form. This herb has high amounts of antioxidants and flavonoids and contains various nutrients like vitamins, calcium, and others. It is perfect for the liver detoxification process. For the capsule-packed, 600-800 take it thrice daily.

Burdock Root

Not the taste you would love, but this root contains antimicrobial blood cleanser, loaded with detoxifying nutrients. Works super-well in washing the liver and lymphatic system. Add dried-up burdock to hot water and allow to strain. Take it as tea once daily.

Multivitamin Tablet

Eat before taking this tablet so that the food will be able to support it in the body. A perfect companion during the detox week.

Probiotics

Probiotics come in different varieties. You can opt for any of the variations. Take at least one capsule per day.

Cilantro

This optional herb is best for heavy metal toxicity. Since this is a powerful herb, you might consider taking it only once during the detox week. Add it to your diluted juices or any other liquid. Consult your medical doctor before making use of Cilantro.

Milk Thistle

Works best in expelling metabolic waste from the body. Take this herb alongside your meals about 2 – 3 times a day.

Liquorice Root

Helps a lot in discarding harmful and poisonous toxic waste from the body system. Simmer for 5 minutes and drink once daily.

Extra Virgin Cold Pressed Organic Oil

Contains fatty acids to help boost the body. This oil can be added to any cooked food during the detox week. Add any quantity you most prefer to your cooked food, so far, the amount does not affect food taste or make it too oily. You may not have to use this oil during Day **4.**

Neem

This herb is also called *Indian Lilac*, and it contains natural blood purifiers. Taking Neem during the detox week helps the body to effectively carry oxygen and several other needed food nutrients around the body. When there is a proper circulation of these food nutrients and oxygen, the liver and kidney area function the way they should. It is best taken as a tea every morning and optionally during other parts of the day.

Ground Ivy

The herb, Ground Ivy helps to expel metallic compounds from the body.

Ginger

Ginger comprises gingerols and shogaols that help to speed up detoxification processes. It helps to wash away toxins from the liver and other body organs and also causes sweat in the process, which aids to move out the toxins.

Pectasol Powder

Pectasol-C® Modified Citrus Pectin provides support for healthy cellular function. This support is due to the mechanisms it comprises of. Apply about 10 – 20 grams of this powder to your diluted fruit juice, smoothies, and other liquid foods.

Related Books to Buy by the Same Author

Dr. Sebi Alkaline Diet Recipe book:

Learn To prepare over 30+ Dr. Sebi Recommended Meals that Naturally Detox the Liver, Reverse Diabetes and High Blood Pressure.

Click Here to Preview and Buy

****

****

Dr. Sebi Diabetes Cure Book:

A Guide on How to Cure Type 2 Diabetes and Reverse High Blood Sugar with Dr. Sebi Approved Herbs and Natural Cure.

Click here to Preview and Buy

****
****

DR. SEBI DIET 101:

A Beginner's Guide on How to Cleanse The Body, Detoxify the Kidney, Liver, Reverse Diabetes and High Blood Pressure, Boost Brain ... Using Dr. Sebi Alkaline Diet Method

Click Here to Preview and Buy

****

****

Dr. Sebi Extended 16 Day Smoothie Detox Guide:

16 Delicious Dr. Sebi Smoothies Recipes for Detox of the Body (liver, kidney), weight loss, better energy, and mental clarity.

Click here to preview and Buy

Made in the USA
Middletown, DE
19 October 2023